ANGRY WOLF

THE STEROID STORIES—
VOLUME ONE

HADA LONGI

authorHOUSE®

AuthorHouse™
1663 Liberty Drive
Bloomington, IN 47403
www.authorhouse.com
Phone: 1 (800) 839-8640

Published by AuthorHouse 08/02/2019

ISBN: 978-1-5462-7871-9 (sc)
ISBN: 978-1-5462-7870-2 (e)

CONTENTS

DEDICATIONS

For those tribe members who have passed on, who are currently too ill to read or think or feel. To the family members and friends who live in the shadow of lupus, this is for you.

Sound Check: *If I Die Young by The Band Perry*

During the writing of this book, my friend, confidant, lover, husband and favorite person, Lafe Brackenridge, Sr. passed away on September 7, 2018. Through everything concerning Lupus and life, he was there. I remember when he shaved his head in solidarity after my hair fell out. He called off work for a week the first time I lost my footing. For those of you who don't have lupus, this means I could not move my legs. I told him about spoon therapy and he came home with a paper bag filled with dollar store spoons. He purchased the laptop I am writing on at this moment. This book is dedicated to his memory.

Sound Check: *See You Again by Wiz Khalifa*

INTRODUCTION

I didn't see the type of things I wanted to see so I did it myself.

– Melvin Van Peebles, How to Eat Your
Watermelon in White Company (and Enjoy It)

The seeds for this piece were sown recently as I spoke to a woman newly diagnosed with discoid Lupus. She just called me out of the blue and we started talking and laughing. I found out later that she was given my phone number from our dermatologist who is the best in the world. She explained that she doesn't really laugh anymore because everything is so serious now. Her family is taking her temperature every 10 minutes, the medication is making her nauseous and she just doesn't have it in her to pretend to be okay anymore.

That's when I decided it's time to talk about the things nobody seems willing to talk about. It's time to take down the wall of privacy and discuss the issues that the doctors don't mention. The issues that are too embarrassing to discuss in 'good' company. Let's face the truth, prednisone makes you hungry and gassy which often makes long distance drives rough.

We are inclined to hide away like hermits. Even at support groups where we should be able to share honestly and openly, we hide. Let's not even talk about the fact that there are cities that still don't have support groups for lupus survivors yet, so this particular group of people are not only isolated but in a state of panic and confusion with nowhere to turn.

Fear not, you are not alone. Do you remember the first time you went to the doctor's office and they pulled out a camera? You're sitting there thinking, "What new hell is this?" The doctor left the room for five minutes and came back with 20 med students and a camera and tells you to get undressed…again; or when you started the new pain meds and started to itch but didn't want to scratch in public because you didn't want people to think you had lice? You scratched anyway, didn't you? Yeah, so did the rest of us, it's all good (I love the new vernacular).

If you can identify with the above paragraph, this book is unquestionably for you. However, if giving your cat a couple of steroids and leaving it in your son's room to play, after telling your son 1000 times to clean the room is problematic for you, well, maybe this is the time for us to part company. I have an extraordinarily vivid imagination and I hate to be bored so I've decided to do things a bit differently.

I'm a huge movie buff and music lover. Unless the movie or song was god-awful (Poltergeist 3 and You Remind Me Of My Jeep), I might make reference to it and that's when you'll see "Sound Check" or "Movie Check." This means, rest your blurry eyes and relax.

For the record, don't expect me to add a lot of disclaimers and excuses to this writing. Life's too short, and my mission is too dire. If you find something offensive, I assume that you have either no sense of humor or you haven't had lupus long enough to actually laugh at yourself and those around you.

In either case, please send any and all hate mail to: Boo Hoo Hoo at: P.O. Box, Get Over It, Clusterfuck, Egypt, 66666. Otherwise, have a good laugh or shed a tear with me. If you are a lupus survivor (tribe member) by all means call me and let's get together for lunch.

Above all else, enjoy the gassy ride!

Sound Check: *Here Comes the Sun by The Beetles*

Allow me to begin by telling you that lupus means 'wolf' in Latin.

I really need to give you a little background information about myself to prove I'm well qualified to speak my mind and go all gangsta about this condition. I'll also give you a very brief overview of the disease itself for people new to our tribe or family members who are still confused. Keep in mind, like I said, it's a brief overview. For more in-depth information, go to the Lupus Foundation of America's website at: www.lupus.org.

I was diagnosed in 1989 by a dermatologist after he did a skin biopsy of a unusual lesion I had on my scalp. My initial diagnosis was discoid lupus - on the skin, but the diagnosis didn't come easy.

Like many of us, I went a long time without being diagnosed and by the time my diagnosis came, I was in crisis mode. Lupus was difficult to find back then. What pissed me off was that I had a couple of doctors who mentioned it in passing like, "you might have lupus, but it's rare, don't worry." Like the butterfly rash wasn't a dead giveaway? I hate stupid people.

No tests were ordered, no referrals to another doctor – nothing! I can't really blame them because let's face it, every doctor wants to make an impact on the world and cure disease. That's why they became doctors in the first place – to heal the world. Many of them will simply walk away from anything attached to the word 'chronic.' I like to refer to this group of physicians as punk-ass M.D's.

Since my initial diagnosis, I crossed over a couple of times to systemic – go figure. Just last week, I went to my rheumatologist "the rheumy" and they couldn't find the lupus antibody in my blood work. One thing's for sure, I've taken great joy over the years at watching my rheumatologists face as he reads my blood work. It's hilarious. He leans back in his chair, sighs and then looks at me over his glasses as I smile at him with the teeth I purchased after having let them suppress my immune system back in 2002. Let's just say it was not one of our greatest decisions or treatments, but at least he tried.

BRIEF OVERVIEW OF LUPUS

Sound Check: *Hungry Like The Wolf by Duran Duran*

Lupus is a widespread and chronic (lifelong) autoimmune disease that, for unknown reasons, causes the immune system to attack the body's own tissue and organs, including the joints, kidneys, heart, lungs, brain (my favorite), blood and skin. This is a limited list because Lupus can affect any organ at any time with a vengeance.

The immune system normally protects the body against viruses, bacteria, and other foreign bodies. In an autoimmune disease like lupus, the immune system loses its ability to tell the difference between foreign substances and its own cells and tissues. The immune system then makes antibodies directed against "self." By that I mean it attacks healthy tissue, not germs.

Lupus is most common in women between the ages of 15 and 44. These are roughly the childbearing years. But don't think for a minute that there are not children who suffer from this condition; I've met quite a few. Anyone can get lupus but African American women are three times more likely to get lupus than white women. It's also more common in Latin and Native American people.

It's becoming more and more prevalent in men, as well. So simply talking to the girls is a thing of the past. Hell, can't we have anything without them ruining it? Think about it – PMS, Putting Up With Men's Shit, menopause, menstruation, hysterectomy and now this. They're even trying to take over breast cancer. I wish I could get a testicular infection Huh, that would show 'em.

Back to being serious, the term lupus was first used to describe red ulcerations on the face. I already told you that the word lupus means wolf and there are two theories as to why it was used.

1) The most common theory is that the skin rash, like a wolf, seemed to eat away the skin and destroy it. The rash, therefore, was said to resemble skin which had actually been bitten by a wolf; and

2) The frightening appearance of some lupus sufferers put people in mind of werewolves. I am not making this up. These were seen as humans who had magical power to transform themselves into animals. The rash was said to make people's faces resemble the face of a wolf and in superstitious middle ages, that meant werewolf.

There's an accurate description of discoid lupus for you. Remember it the next time someone stares at you on the street. Growl and run in the opposite direction. That'll fix their little red wagon.

Today, there are three types of lupus. I've been hearing rumors of another but haven't been able to find any factual documentation on it so, I'll leave it out or add it next time.

1) Discoid (cutaneous) lupus is always limited to the skin and is identified by a rash that may appear on the face, neck and scalp. Discoid lupus accounts for approximately 10% to 20% of all cases.

2) Systemic lupus is usually more severe than discoid lupus, and can affect any organ or system of the body. Approximately 60% of lupus cases are systemic. In about half of these cases, major organs will be affected.

3) Drug-induced lupus occurs after use of certain prescribed drugs. The symptoms of drug-induced lupus are similar to systemic lupus. The drugs most commonly connected with drug-induced lupus are used to treat high blood pressure or used to treat heart arrhythmia. The percentage of individuals using these drugs who develop drug-induced lupus is extremely small, and the symptoms usually fade when the medications are discontinued.

People are talking about pregnancy induced lupus but most of the documentation agrees that pregnancy just awakens the beast but does not create it.

Symptoms

- Symptoms of lupus often mimic other less serious illnesses.

- Symptoms can range from mild to life-threatening.
- Joint pain, swelling and stiffness, skin rashes, photosensitivity, patchy areas of hair loss or complete hair loss (alopecia), dry eyes and dry mouth, kidney inflammation, low white blood cell count, blood clotting problems, etc.

Some of the more life-threatening or danger signs are: Wait! Before I go on, if anyone reading this is experiencing any of these symptoms, see your doctor right away. Put this damn book down and call immediately. Do not wait.

- Severe chest pain, severe shortness of breath, especially if accompanied by sudden chills or a temperature of 101.5, difficulty speaking or jumbled words, severe headaches, fainting, seizures, sudden swelling of feet and ankles, weakness or numbness of arms, legs or in my case face and extreme fatigue.

These are almost all of the symptoms I was having at work. One day, I couldn't even scream for help from my co-worker across the hall. I should have known I was dog meat but not me. Naw. The brain is a funny organ.

I'm going to say this one more time to be clear because I can't stress it enough. If you've been suffering over a period of time from any of the symptoms I've put on my critical list, get to the doctor's office immediately.

Once you get there, demand that the doctor test you for lupus. Say whatever you have to say, fall out in the floor, make yourself vomit, I don't care. Demand an ANA (antinuclear antibody test) by name. Feel no shame. Finding out if you have lupus can be one of the hardest things you ever do because there is no test that you can take that's specific to lupus.

The test results could very well come back negative, but you could also be saving your own life. My position is, if they can test you for AIDS they can test you for lupus too. And if they refuse to test you for any reason, call the Lupus Foundation. We will start a letter and phone campaign that will make you proud to know us. Hell, I'll call the doctor my damn self if need be. I've been trying to grind this axe for a long time.

Diagnosis

Making a diagnosis of lupus can be difficult because the symptoms can develop so slowly that no pattern emerges, or they come and go. Symptoms have disappeared by the time the individual has seen their physician. Time and a lot of patience are required for both physician and patient.

A definite diagnosis is based on:

- A detailed medical history.
- A thorough physical exam, in which the physician looks for any signs and symptoms suggestive of lupus.
- Various blood tests, which gives cell counts, immunological information and looks for the presence of antinuclear antibodies.

- Lastly, other diseases with similar lab results to Systemic Lupus Erythmatosis or SLE must be ruled out.
- Lab tests like the ANA which measures the amount of antibody detected in the blood that corresponds with how active lupus is, along with skin or kidney biopsies. The biopsies may not be necessary, particularly if the blood work comes back positive.

In my case, the blood work came back negative but the skin biopsy was positive. Remember this was in the late 80's so they were really perplexed by me.

If either or all of your tests come back positive you will normally need to see a rheumatologist. They specialize in treating diseases that affect the joints and muscles, like lupus. Your dermatologist should work hand in hand with your rheumy if you're diagnosed with discoid.

Treatment

Treatment is tailored to the needs of each individual and is based on the type and severity of the symptoms. As the disease waxes and wanes so does the treatment require changing.

Arthritis or arthritis like symptoms are a common thread with lupus. We all hurt at some point. Mild can be treated with a non Rx, over the counter pain medication. If inflammation does not subside, there are several other medications that can be used to control this condition.

But as you know, every medication has its downside. Therefore, people who take medication should become knowledgeable about possible side effects and report any difficulties immediately to their doctor. Doctors prefer to use the least powerful medication for the shortest period of time required to bring symptoms under control.

Coping with lupus

Every patient is different. My arm may hurt today and your ears may ring. There are no identical lupus patients. We all need to find out what works for us. We'll discuss this further in a later chapter.

People with lupus have limited energy and have to manage it wisely. School and work are difficult but it can be done. I did it for a very long time. So can you, just don't overdo it like I did. Pace yourself.

We have to stay out of the sun and if it's absolutely necessary to go out, try avoiding it between the hours of noon and 4:00pm. Don't forget to use sun block and protective clothing at all times. I've failed miserably at this task. I love camping and outdoor sports so even after all these years I try to wear sun block. Finding one that doesn't make me itch is hard. Plus, when we go kayaking or canoeing, it's really uncomfortable to be wet and completely covered with sunblock. The new ones are actually quite helpful and don't make you feel like you're being weighed down by drywall mud.

I love to hike and after about 25 minutes the long sleeves end up around my waist. I was born and raised in Atlantic City, NJ and no matter where I am, I need to find a beach from time to time to reenergize. It's almost like a spiritual connection to the ocean. My dad once told me that anyone who grew up on the Jersey Shore needs to come home from time to time to feel the sand between their toes and regroup.

Don't make your life complicated. Go online and check out clothes for people with photosensitivity. A couple of on-line stores that I use are:

www.sungrubbies.com and www.coolibar.com

There are more but these are the two I find reliable. Happy hunting!

One last thing before I end this chapter. It's very difficult to deal with a chronic illness, particularly one that's so mysterious and crippling. Some of us go into a state of absolute denial followed by a long period of mourning before we can come to terms with this disease. We need to be surrounded by people who care.

Compassion and education is better than all the medication in the world, which is why everyone needs to be educated about this disease.

And should anyone say, "You don't look sick," punch them in the face and "low run" away like Lon Chaney in The Wolfman.

TRIBE MEMBERS

No!! You are not crazy, it's the steroids. Yeah, maybe you've driven past your own house a few times before you realized where the hell you were going. So what your left shoe is in the freezer. It happens to us all at one point on this journey.

The word lupus is synonymous with steroid. Nine times out of ten, if you have lupus, you are or will be on a steroid at some point in your life. Relax and enjoy the ride. Don't panic. You'll probably have a really good doctor, like the one I have who will take you off of it unless your symptoms are severe.

Tell anyone that questions your weight gain or pie face that you're studying to become the first U.S. sumo wrestler and you need to buff up. Don't forget to go online and research what a sumo wrestler is. It works for me and people are in awe.

What really used to startle me when I would tell people that I had lupus was that everyone who I told would say the same thing. They didn't mean any harm, they were just uninformed. They all say they had a friend or relative to die from this disease. The purpose of this writing is to let everyone know that this condition is not an automatic death sentence. We have to start sharing information within our ranks and disseminating information to the public that is accurate and responsible. We also need to laugh more. That's where I come in.

Recently, while at a doctor's appointment, I heard the most brilliant thing. I was chatting with another tribe member in the waiting area and she said that she has separated her closet. One side is for when she's on the steroids and the other is for when she's off. What I heard her say was that on one side she keeps her size 8 pants and on the other, her size 16. I never thought of that before. I just throw everything in together. There's a nugget of information you didn't ask for. See, the 'roids are kicking in and now I'm writing random shit.

Memory Loss and Prednisone Moments

Here's a movie that covers both memory loss and steroids. Pay attention to the Sean Astin's character on 'roids. It's classic.

Movie Check: *50 First Dates by Adam Sandler*

Don't beat yourself up about the small stuff. Life is too short. Shake it off and keep it moving forward. Memory loss and absence of thought are a very common problem that we have. Embrace it. You might one day look back and find that those were the best days of all. If nothing else, the most entertaining.

Mental impairments are common with lupus. We need to come to terms with this elusive aspect of our elusive disease. Many of our tribe members suffer from subtle, but insidious losses in critical mental functions as memory, information processing and concentration.

We are not going to spend the next hour discussing nerve cell receptors or the cerebral cortex of the brain or even how certain receptors bind the neurotransmitter glutamate so let's start our ride.

I remember picking my daughter up from school and missing the turn off to our house. She says, "Where are we going?" I looked over at her like *she* was the crazy one and said, "Home." I mean, what kind of question is that? We come home the same way every day. Being the smart ass 13 year olds tend to be, she then replies in classic teen fashion, "Did we move?"

I kind of shake the fog off and realize I've driven two blocks too far. Now I'm embarrassed so not to miss a beat, I tell her since she's been so wonderful that week, I decided to take her to McDonalds for a treat. Sounds good right? I played it off superbly. It would have been perfect had I not missed the same damn turn going back home. Shit happens.

My favorite all-time laugh at myself moment came one Monday afternoon as I was preparing to go grocery shopping. I was talking to my husband to see if he wanted anything particular from the grocery store. As we're talking, I'm getting myself together to walk out of the house, ya know – keys, wallet, etc. I go into the bathroom, put my 'hair' on and I'm ready to go. All that's left to do is find my keys and cell phone. I'm searching the living room for my keys but no cell phone. I'm starting to panic and my husband asks me what's wrong. I tell him I can't find my cell phone. He bursts into playful laughter and said, "have you checked your ear?" Y'all, I was talking to him on my cell phone the entire time I was looking for the thing.

Try not to make the same mistakes I made and you might get through it without looking like an ass, or by all means, take the Hada approach and have fabulous stories to tell your grandchildren.

Sound Check: I'm Sorry by The Platters

We used to have Christmas parties every year when the kids were growing up. Nothing much, sometimes it was a pot-luck, sometimes we'd just feed people. We'd buy beer, wine, etc. and call our friends and say, "come on over." We were very informal about it and kids were always invited.

Well, one year things weren't going so well for me and as you know, when you start taking steroids, you can get emotional. One moment you're laughing, the next you're in tears. I started on about 50 mgs twice a day, which for me is a lot. 100 mgs in all, folks. Let the show begin.

I had spent days apologizing for putting my foot in my mouth or doing things that no one understood but I was resolved to press on.

It's day three and I've been on this high dosage for at least three weeks. People started crowding into our house. Let's face it, our friends loved to come over - always good drama at our house. I'm feeling weird but I'm ready. We're all talking and laughing and drinking and smoking and yelling – you know the type of party: intimate. Suddenly, one of my husband's best friends says something that I, for reasons I will never understand, find annoying and discourteous.

What do I do as the polite, sophisticated, wonderful hostess? Do I redirect the conversation? Noooo. Do I offer more libation to the guests or refill anyone? Nooo! I jump out of my seat and announce to the entire party that I think this guy is a butt reaming asshole living in a "sack of dicks." Yes, I really said it and yes, the children were present. The room is now quiet enough to hear people blink and everyone is staring at me. My husband, being my defender say's "don't pay her any mind. It's the 'roids."

The room cracked up.

My favorite 'can't wait to tell the grandkids story' also happened at one of our Christmas parties. The 13 year old was about three and I forgot that tannins, a substance found in red wine, does not mix well with steroids. Glass three, I see my daughter in the living room playing with my friends son, Keven. She's chasing him and he's running from her. It was kind of sweet, really. He was 13 and showing love to the baby.

I'm checking out the room feeling blessed to have these people in our lives when all of a sudden, I look up and see her run towards Keven, who is not paying attention. In the blink of an eye, she runs towards him and he unintentionally side steps.

Before she can stop herself, she hits the wall flat and bounces half way across the living room, lands on her back and is motionless for at least 3 seconds.

My husband hurls his body out of his chair and rushes to her side. The other children begin to cry and there is absolute pandemonium in the room. I will never forget Keven's face for as long as I live. He was devastated. My husband grabs our daughter and hurriedly reaches for the phone.

What do I do? Me, the woman who has shot flames from her eyes over her children; the woman who has suffered the stigmata over a high fever? I burst into uproarious laughter and accidentally peed a little.

I know in my heart that if he thought he could have gotten away with it, my husband would have killed me and buried me under the house without blinking an eye. He shot me a look that I felt in the pit of my soul. My girlfriend is kneeling next to him now by this child's side, looks from me to him and say's loudly, "the 'roids?" He nods.

She wiggles out of her father's arms and runs to me screaming. I grab her and try to look at her face. I can't see through my own tears of laughter, but I notice, what we call in South Jersey, a visible 'water knot' beginning to grow directly in the middle of her forehead.

I'm trying to comfort and sooth this precious child when all of a sudden she announces to the party that I smell like pee. My secret was out. My brother, trying to be helpful say's, "well you scared your mom and she had an accident."

Even at three years old, this kid had an amazing sense of humor and reply's, "Nu uh, she was laughing at me, again" and starts to giggle. Everyone looks amazed. My husband puts the phone down and is on his hands and knees, bless his heart, looking like he's having a heart attack, while she sits on my lap laughing with me.

The moral of these stories should be, don't drink on your 'roids, I guess. But that's not it at all. The moral of these stories is that we're full of medication. It comes out in bizarre ways sometimes and the only thing we can do is attempt to process it, ask for forgiveness and forgive ourselves. Be gentle. I've got a million dumb-ass things that I have done. Those pesky neurotransmitters.

Ummm…before you call child protective services or label me a terrible mother, understand that she was fine and I took her to the pediatrician the very next morning and told the entire story to the doctor just like I'm telling you guys. Guess what she did? Yup, she laughed her ass off.

We no longer have yearly Christmas parties but if we decide to resume the tradition, you'll get an invitation.

Appearance

Movie Check: *Now Voyager, Betty Davis*

Quick sidebar: You have got to purchase this movie – my wolf commands it! I never knew that I might have lesbian tendencies until I saw poor "Aunt Charlotte" walk off that cruise ship. I *always* have her in mind when I have the opportunity to play dress-up and go out. Her suit was magnificent, her shoes fabulous and her hat to die for.

When I'm feeling like that, I always listen to:

Sound Check: *The Men All Pause by Klymaxx*

Everyone wants to look their best. We go all out for makeup supplies, clothes, hair gel, shoes, the works. We want to smell good and put our best foot forward. We want to be fabulous and why not? When I put my 'street' face on, far more people want to chat with me. When I'm in the inflammation zone and not wearing anything but sunshine on my face people tend to avoid me.

Gather 'round, all ye discoid lupus tribe members. I have two words for you to remember: Fuck them. Make these two little words your mantra and you can't go wrong. Make no mistake; it took me a long, long, long, time to be able to come to terms with this thing so I know what I'm talking about. First off, the people who love you are just happy you're alive so don't worry about them. They love you no matter what. Love them back in the best way you can.

I think this might be a good time to describe myself to you. Here's what I need you to do. Go to the grocery store and purchase an ice cream bar. Get the kind that has vanilla on the inside and hard chocolate on the outside. Try to get the ones that have the little curvy thingy at the very top.

Now, very gently take your teeth and bite around the top. Be careful because if you bite too hard, the chocolate coating on the outside will break and the flat side will begin to slide off and we don't want that. Okay, now take your teeth and very gently expose just the top of the ice cream. You should have a white top and a chocolate bottom.

Look at it and say, "it's nice to meet you." Please be polite. I hate rude people. Without makeup and hair, you are looking at me. My lupus comes with lots of cool prizes. One of them is vitiligo. It's a loss of melanin in the skin. Michael Jackson said it was the reason he bleached. But people like me know that it's genetic and other people in his family would have had it, if his story was legit. My vitiligo is from the neck up. Seriously, you can see where it begins.

It runs in our family but used to skip a generation until I came along. Another of my really cool prizes is alopecia universalis - a complete loss of body hair. Well except for my left eye lashes. I never quite figured out why I have no eye brows or lashes, but I have a very healthy set of hair on my left eye. Go figure. Oh, and feel free to eat the ice cream now before it melts. I was going to say "eat me" but well, that's rude.

I used to hate it when people stared. I avoided eye contact because I was embarrassed and ashamed of the way I looked. There was no covering it when I was active so I'd have to compose myself before doing everyday activities like grocery shopping. You should check me out now. I go straight for the eyes and say, "is there something you need?"

The worse was having kids stare, point and whisper while their parents did nothing. Maybe they don't think we know how we look but we know how we look. While transitioning, I looked brown with white speckles. I can't speak for you but my mother taught us early in the game not to stare. Pointing was out of the question unless you wanted a nice double whack or as my children call it, a 'two piece" with a biscuit. We don't do rude in this house.

My children know that beauty is only skin deep but ugly is to the bone. And if you're ugly on the inside, you're ugly on the outside. Thank God we had these discussions before the discoid blew out of control so they know it's a fact of life and not just me justifying my own appearance.

I know I'm going to catch all manner of hell, but I have to tell you this. I had a relative who, like the rest, shall remain nameless. Supermodel gorgeous. She would walk into a room and heads would turn. She was tall, a little overweight, funny and sexy as all get out. She always had her makeup kit, comb and brush to keep her perm together and everything she needed to be and stay beautiful until 4 am. Sista had it going on and I loved her for it. She made us proud and may she rest in eternal peace.

Sound Check: *Beauty's Only Skin Deep by The Temptations*

The problem with her was that every time she saw me or anyone else who wasn't absolutely fabulous, she'd sneer and look at them like they stank and make suggestions. You know the type. You look fat in that. You need to wear heals. Why don't you wear makeup? You need to do something about this or that, or with your hair and your children's hair. A couple of my kids decided to wear their hair in dreadlocks and she thought it was a hell worthy tresspass that I didn't perm their hair.

What she didn't remember was that time and tide wait for no man. Beauty fades and if you don't have a pleasing disposition or a whole lot of money, you're going to leave this world feeling pretty damn disappointed. My kids showed me a picture of her on Facebook and I swear to God, I had to ask them who it was. I didn't even recognize her. All I saw was an old, tired looking woman.

Give your significant other a big shout out for knowing what's really important. And appreciate that the beautiful pointers and haters are going to grow old one day. Time marches on and eventually it will march across your face. As a matter of fact, go give your friends a big squeeze if you can. They know what true beauty is and where it comes from.

Where was I? Oh well, it doesn't matter.

What bothered my husband when we went out was that as I was going about my business doing whatever, people were gawking at me. I was paying no attention to them, but he had the privilege of seeing their faces as they stared at me. I've seen him almost go to blows about it. My children would look at other children with a look like, "what the fuck are you staring at?" It's not just about you. Lupus really is a family disease. So make it a point of having regular discussions with your family. Listen to them. Let them know you understand how they feel and why. Encourage them to attend support groups and spend your bail money on a fabulous scarf.

As for you, keep your damn head up. Don't walk down the street looking at your shoes with a big ass, over-sized hoodie, or scarf trying not to be seen. Shake your shimmies with your head held high with your sexy-ass red floppy hat. Don't let it get you down. Worrying about it is the worst thing we can do. Hell, stress has killed more people than cancer so what would be the point?

What does not kill you makes you either pissed off or makes you stronger. It will allow you to one day giggle as you sit in front of your laptop and write about how your head looks like a boiled egg with eyes. It will make you become a 7 year old again and put your husband's shirt on your head and swing it around like Cher every time you see a shampoo commercial. And if anyone says anything to you about it, get out your ice cream bar. You know, the one that looks like me and say, "eat me" without blinking an eye.

What is our mantra? Fuck them.

Sound Check: *Miss Celie's Blues, The Color Purple*

Religion

Movie Check: *Dogma by Kevin Smith*

Relax. My parents taught me as a small child during the Nixon administration that arguing religion and politics is futile. That's not where I'm at. I'm just talking about myself and the issues that I feel are funny. Experiences that I've had that you might relate to and even appreciate. See what I did there? I redirected you. I told you I'm good like that.

When I first found out that I had lupus, I was completely and utterly devastated. Like many of you I'm certain, I went into a total and complete state of denial. I walked around like I was perfectly normal. The nothing is wrong, all is well, thank you for asking, brand of normal.

I got up every morning, got the kids together for school, went to work, picked the kids up, went home, cooked dinner, read books to the kids, prepared for the next day and forced myself to think of every and anything except lupus.

I was raised a good Missionary Baptist girl. I was saved (at the time) and "He who the savior has set free, is free indeed." I remember talking to church folk and having them tell me that since I looked good, the doctors obviously didn't know what they were talking about so, "don't speak it into existence." If anyone says that to you, I want you to turn around and open hand slap the hell out of them. They deserve it and yeah, you can blame it on the 'roids.

After a few years, as the condition began to progress I started searching for my roots, you know? Something to suspect that if you've had this disease for more than a couple of years and have had your share of "flares" you know what I'm talking about. You are or were reaching for something that the doctors don't have. Spending long, painful, endless nights trying to figure out what you did to deserve such a terrible fate.

Rummaging around in the trashcan of your memory trying to remember what crimes against God or your fellow man you had committed so you could apologize, repent and be healed.

True story. One night I had just experienced a major flare and was in tears. Everything hurt. The inflammation was so bad that the pain medication would not and could not take effect. Fellow tribe members, I was a sick puppy that night and desperate.

"The children were nestled all snug in their beds, while visions of sugar plums danced in their heads." My little people had been asleep for hours and my husband was snoring. The house was quiet and now was my chance.

If any one of y'all Baptist or Pentecostal people laugh, I will hunt you down and kick your ass. Tribe, I went into the closet. An actual closet. It was one of those ashes and sack cloth moments y'all, so stop laughing. My mother used to say that sometimes prayer and supplication were the way out of a stew and that's what I was in…a stew.

I knew in my heart I was doing the right thing because first of all, my large, prednisone filled ass and stomach actually fit in the closet.

Well, alright. I'm on my painful knees, in a dark closet with the door shut and I begin to pray, "Dear Lord, Master of the Universe, my Morning Star, my Alpha and Omega, my Light, my Comforter, and my Miracle Worker. I praise Your name." Suddenly I became the great gospel singer, Edna Tatum. "I am speaking to the One that deferred the council of the Holy Trinity and organized an angelic host to furnish music while the glory of Your Father, flooded the hills of Bethlehem, stepped on a heavenly made airplane and rode down through a low ground of sorrow. Leaped into the Virgin Mary and was born one day, in the city of David, wrapped in swaddling clothes and laid in a manger…"

I prayed for rain in the Sudan and peace in the sovereign country of Jackson, Mississippi. I know in my heart that if any demons were around for the first half hour, by minute 45, they were like, "awww, hell no! This is bullshit, we out!" and fled.

Y'all don't hear me. I prayed my house right down to the ground. When I was done, I knew beyond a shadow of a doubt that all was going to be right with the world. I think I may have even started humming because, humming, as we Baptist have been taught, confuses the devil. What I didn't know was that I had been in that damn closet shouting.

I'm tired, my mouth is dry and I've got to be to work by 8:30 but mission accomplished. I open the closet door and look up to find three little faces just staring down at me with eyes wide as saucers. I don't need to tell you what happened next. They laughed at me and my husband never stopped snoring.

Today, I attend a church that works for me. They don't give me judgmental looks when they haven't seen me in a while and seem authentically pleased to see me when I do. They immediately embraced my children and supported my family from day one. We are Unitarian Universalists and we love it. I knew the first time I walked through those big doors at All Souls, Unitarian Universalist Church, here in Washington, DC that I was home and I was safe and that God heard me pray in the closet that night.

The point that I'm trying to make is that you'll begin to understand that there might be a power greater than yourself. Call it what you want: God, The Creator, Spirit of Life, whatever. Illness brings everyone to a certain spiritual level. Some of us turn away from religion and spirituality completely. That's not my story but no judgement here.

We are all here for a reason, so don't feel sorry for yourself. Have you taken the time to think that maybe lupus *is* your reason for being on the planet? Huh, have you? Maybe it's your sacred duty to go forth and preach the 'gospel' of lupus in order to help others cope with this condition? Your pity-pot ain't goin' anywhere and will be in the house when you get back from your mission. I'll take the time to throw you a pity party myself and bring wine and cheese.

Many of us can honestly say we're more like Madea in the Tyler Perry movies when she said, "I haven't prayed since the last time I saw flashing lights in my rear view mirror." You begin to find a certain calm in simply knowing that you're not alone. And believe me, you're not.

FYI, God and I have spoken to one another recently and we sincerely love one another. We have, however, decided to see other people from time to time. Oh, shut up! You know it's funny.

TAKING CONTROL OF YOUR HEALTH

Let's talk 'real.' Don't get this section twisted. I am a wellness consultant by trade so I'm really serious about this. I am under no circumstances suggesting that your doctor is crazy. I am not giving medical advice or trying to encourage you to stop taking your medication or start a new one. I am not *your* consultant. I am a member of the tribe.

I started writing this with discoid lupus in mind so there is a lot of information about the skin.

Every lupus patient is different. Some of us decided that we'd take extra measure in our attempt to feel better. What worked for me, may not work for you. My results have been through trial and error. I think information is power but don't put yourself at risk. Speak with your doctor before starting or stopping any treatment. Are we clear? Good, let's start by discussing medical marijuana…

Weed

Sound Check: *Pusher Man by Curtis Mayfield*

One word: remarkable. It has taken me over 20 years to understand why people are screaming at local government and congress about the legalization of marijuana. Just recently, I was with another discoid lupus tribe member and I was telling her that I was having a hard time controlling the pain again. It wasn't so much the lupus; it was just me being me. I got lazy and let my routine slip.

Actually, it was a combination of lupus, PMS, bad diet (because of PMS) and constipation (because of bad diet). It's a vicious circle. Anyway, I was in HALT mode: hungry, angry, lonely and tired.

Sound Check: *PMS by Mary J. Blige*

My face was so red, it looked like I had been slapped about 10 times on both sides of my face. That's a dead giveaway that my condition is active. I get all red, inflamed and bumpy. Sometimes my skin hurts and burns when touched. It feels like I have sunburn but there is no relief. I can't shower because the water beating on my skin hurts. I do wash though, so don't make fun. Sometimes I can only wear cotton because any other material irritates my skin. Mens shirts are a God send.

By the way, if your skin hurts or burns like mine does sometimes, you might want to try using those nifty little wipes made by Ponds. They also make cold cream but those wipes clean and moisturize like nobody's business. I definitely keep them on hand for the tough days. So yeah, I'm clean, punk.

I'm telling my friend about the night I had and she, in perfect form, pulls out a perfectly rolled joint. It was machine rolled perfect like a cigarette. Don't ask me why but I started looking around and giggling like a 16 year old. I hadn't seen a joint for an awful long time and never one like this.

I jumped up (the 'roids), and shut my bedroom door and said, "what the hell are you doing?" She said, "trust me." She fires up a joint and I'm listening to make sure nobody's coming. I should tell you that we were alone in my house. I'm just thinking, we have crossed a line. We begin to smoke. A couple hours and bags of chips later she say's "go look at your face." I promise you, there was no redness to be seen. I was able to take over the counter Motrin for the pain and slept like a baby that night.

Why? What we know is that marijuana helps with nausea associated with chemo. We know that it helps with vision problems associated with glaucoma and can be used to abate a host of other conditions. What I didn't know was that it helps reduce inflammation and once the inflammation is under control, pain medication can begin to work. You might not even need pain meds.

I am not telling you to leave home seeking your nearest street corner pharmaceutical sales and marketing rep. I'm saying, talk with your doctor and discuss the possibility of using a natural herb or pharmaceutical grade marijuana. Let the "just say no" guys suffer through the pain. We certainly don't deserve to. If your state has yet to legalize cannabis, start the petition and let the rest of us know so we can sign and do everything in our power to help.

Alcohol

Sound Check: *Why Don't We Get Drunk by Jimmy Buffett*

I laugh and tease a lot about my wine drinking but don't get me wrong. It's very easy to turn a harmless bottle of wine into a 28 day stint in rehab. The reason I want to bring this up is because it's an issue you don't read about in your monthly lupus update magazine.

You have no idea what a problem this can become if you're sitting around feeling sorry for yourself. You can easily find yourself sitting alone at home with a glass of alcohol in one hand the television remote in the other at 9:30 in the morning thinking everything is copacetic.

I've been lucky enough to dodge this bullet but I know several tribe members who were not so lucky. It's a problem that we don't talk about. You're sick and think you can do what you want. This is not the way to go. Imagine detoxifying from alcohol and steroids at the same time. That's what they make you do in rehab. Scared yet? I'm scared for you.

Last month I met a new tribe member online and she wanted to get together. After we talked on the phone for a few minutes she said "let's get together for happy hour. Do you drink?" Without waiting for me to answer, she said "you have lupus, of course you drink."

We both laughed because she might be right but what surprised me was that, like me, she had met her share of drunken werewolves. I suspect that part of the problem is self-esteem and the need to hide somewhere safe. Believe me, the bottom of a bottle of alcohol is not a good place to hide. It's like the kid we knew growing up who would hide behind a skinny tree or light post while playing hide and seek. You're not hiding, you're just making others laugh by doing stupid shit.

We, your fellow tribe members, know all too well the feelings of isolation and impending doom that is associated with both SLE and discoid lupus. We understand what it's like to use excuses and diversions in order to never leave the house or attempt to lock yourself away. We feel you! We are you! We look for doubt and dishonesty in our family's eyes and question the motives of our friends. And some of us drink to hide the pain.

You are beautiful, intelligent and worthy of love. My problem is that I can't love you until you love yourself. If you're sitting around telling people that your 'not at think as we drink you are,' I have one thing to say. "Quit that shit right now." Go find something important to do like volunteer at your local lupus center. Hang around like minded people (not drunks) and you will eventually see your way clear.

If you think you've already crossed the bridge into full blown alcoholism, find the nearest A.A. meeting and stay there. Keep going back. They say it works if you work it. It really does.

Has anyone seen my glass of wine?

Lifestyle and Nutrition

Movie Check: *Diet For A New America by John Robbins*

There is a direct correlation, between diet and symptoms. Lupus can be controlled and I went at it full force. Like I said its trial and error. I searched so much that I ended up becoming a wellness consultant. I am a Graduate of The Ekaya Institute of Living Food Education (E.I.L.F.E.), Certified Nutrition Specialists, Raw Living Foods Chef, Raw Lifestyle Coach, and Raw Personal Trainer.

I started slow and below you'll find an example of how I went about it. I remember feeling a little dumb at first but that desperation kicked in and I moved forward. It took me about 4-6 months to go completely raw but after eating vegan (no meat or dairy) I was ready. I'm adding a few facts for those who are curious about it.

A major benefit that I found is that it helps with my energy level and thought patterns. I don't blank as much when I'm eating raw and/or organic. The slow but steady exercise helps loosen my joints and water keeps me hydrated. When I say slow and steady, I mean lying in bed arching my back or attempting leg lifts without screaming in pain. If you are capable of other exercise, get to it. Some of us are slow out of the gate. I think I'd be in so much more pain if this wasn't part of my plan and I am afraid to test the theory.

I cheat from time to time. Particularly when I'm taking the steroids because then I crave red meat and wine. But otherwise, I try to stay away from meat, dairy and on good days, cooked food altogether. No one's perfect but taking tiny steps is better than nothing. You decide.

Why eat raw?

- It is the food nature designed for us to eat, and nature is a very accurate and precise designer!
- Nutrients die at 150 degrees of heat so when you eat cooked food it can't nourish you!
- Try it for one day and you will feel incredible!
- Try it for one year and you will look and feel at least a decade younger!

What do raw foodists eat? Everything! I make a fabulous sunflower seed pate' with avocado, lettuce, tomato and any other veggie I can get my hands on. My family loves it.

What happens when we change our diet?
Your body will detoxify, which may cause temporary flu-like symptoms. I recommend a transition diet schedule: one month vegetarian (no meat), one month vegan (no meat or dairy), one month raw with one cooked meal a day (raw food and a meal such as rice and steamed vegetables), one month raw with one cooked meal a week, and then 90% raw/20% vegan, eating mostly whole foods with some simple 100% raw whole food recipes.

Fruit Salad
1 avocado, 2 bananas, 1 mango. Chop, mix, and enjoy this texture blend from paradise!

Cleansing Citrus Salad

4 oranges - peeled, 2 grapefruit – peeled, 2 tablespoons agave nectar

Cut oranges and grapefruit in half, remove seeds and pull apart each section. If grapefruit skin is tough, separate from pulp and discard. Add agave nectar and mix well.

Spinach Salad

1 pound spinach – stems removed, 2 garlic cloves – sliced thin, ¼ cup fresh lemon juice, ¼ cup extra virgin olive oil, 1 tomato – sliced and quartered, ¼ brown olives – pitted and sliced.

Wash and massage spinach, mix with remaining ingredients. Share with someone.

If it's something you think you might be interested in, email me. The tribe members that have gone this route, rarely go back to eating 100% cooked food and cheat from time to time but try to stay away from meat and dairy because it makes us feel better when we eat lighter. There is actually scientific precedent for this, but if I go deeply into it you'll hear Charlie Browns teacher and I'm not trying to bore you to tears.

Relaxation

Music Check: Whatever works for you – just don't listen to gangsta rap.

Movie Check: Whatever calms you – just don't watch *Eat, Pray, Love*. I know I can't possibly be the only person that wanted to scratch their own eyes out after watching that movie. Where does the average human being find the cash to just up and go to Bali? But I digress...

Stress can impede your thought processes and hamper your thinking. You may find making simple decisions like what to have for dinner or remembering directions to a restaurant are more difficult when you're stressed out.

People dealing with chronic stress may be easily frustrated and quick to lose their temper. They may cry more often and spend considerably more time worrying. This we can't completely blame on the steroids but the medication can play a part.

Strange as it may seem, stress can take a toll on your oral health, which is why the dentist is considering removing ALL of my teeth. In terms of its effect on the body, stress is dangerous to your heart. Stress hormones speed up your heart rate, constrict blood vessels, and make the heart and blood vessels more likely to overreact in the event of a future stressful event. Stress is also linked to high blood pressure, blood clots, and even stroke.

Stress may make skin problems such as psoriasis, eczema, acne, discoid lupus and rosacea worse. Your hair may begin to fall out. When a person is under a great deal of stress, his or her hair may enter the falling-out stage of the hair life cycle. Hair usually grows back within a year unless you have discoid lupus and the follicles die like in my case.

Most of us are already feeling sick. It may be because your stress is suppressing your already suppressed immune system, making you more susceptible to infection. Stress can worsen symptoms of chronic illness such as rheumatoid arthritis, diabetes and lupus.

Is it really worth it? Lie back on your bed and clear your head (it even rhymes). Turn on whatever music moves you and relax. Diffuse essential oils like Citrus Fresh or Grapefruit and clear your mind.

Think about me. Ponder the mysteries of the universe. Have a good belly laugh. Think about this: How does Cee Lo Green wipe his ass? His arms look too short to reach around so does he come from the front or does he pay someone to do it for him. How much does he pay to have someone wipe him and is it a full time job. Whatever you need to do, just let go of the stress.

Let the Sun Shine

Sound Check: *Soak Up the Sun by Sheryl Crow*

Just keep it out of your face. It's not your imagination. You really are melting. I spoke earlier about how much I love being outside but not anymore. I'm now the one watching the weather channel waiting for an over cast day.

I don't care if I *am* the one assigned to bring beer to the cook-out, if it's a mid-day event, I'm going to be late. Get over it. You knew before you asked, and I don't drink beer anyway. I only said yes because…STOP! Cee Lo Green, Cee Lo Green…

Wow. That was weird but I'm now stress free.

My family and I are going to Los Angeles for 2 ½ weeks and we're making plans to hit it hard. We'll stay in LA for a few days hanging with my husband's family and friends. He hasn't been home in over ten years so we can't complain. We'll hang out with family in Vegas and party. After he's visited out, we're renting a convertible and driving to San Diego for a couple days. The plan is to drive from San Diego, up the coast to San Francisco, across the Golden Gate Bridge, and back to LA through the mountains with the top down. The drive of a lifetime.

This is how I know my family wants me dead. But for every problem, there is a solution. I'm strategizing now and coming up with creative ways to be part of this adventure without being hospitalized before we get out of Vegas.

What would 'Aunt Charlotte' do? She'd find fabulous hats and scarves to wear. She'd load up on sun block to protect her, oh-so delicate skin. She'd search for sexy clothes that protect her from the sun, yet make her butt look marvelous. And that's what I'm going to do. Having fun and looking good count. Being safe is even more important. Depending on the heat, my precious 13 year old may end up riding up the coast with a vampire friendly sedan with the air condition on. I ain't dying for her.

Trust me, it's not worth getting sick over. If you absolutely, positively have to be in the sun, protect yourself at all times. No matter what.

FAMILY

Sometimes your family and friends are so close to you that, as the saying goes, they 'can't see the forest for the trees.' They lose their ability to be objective. They love you and hate your disease which can feel a lot like they are hating on you. That's not usually the case, though.

Sometimes their anger at the disease may be expressed as though it were directed at you personally. Don't be angry with them. They just feel helpless and scared.

All you need to do is cuss them out and blame it on the 'roids the next day.

Movie Check: *Claudine with James Earl Jones, Diahann Carroll*

Like many of you, I have a family. My family consists of 3 daughters, a son and a husband I often refer to as their father. Actually, he has been a good dad but there are times I'd like to bury him in the yard. Fortunately for him, I'm too exhausted most of the time to even bother.

For instance, he came home from work one day and say's "why is the house *still* a wreck?" Truthfully, that's not what he said. His actual words were more along the lines of "why didn't you clean the damn house today?" Yup! That's really what he said to his poor, drunken, lupus suffering wife. My smart-ass response was, "because I spent the day looking for my pubic hair." I thought it was clever. This bastard comes back with, "well I hope like hell you found it because I haven't even seen a pube in about 4 months." Okay, maybe I should have given my answer a little thought before I let it pop out of my mouth but still…low blow. I wanted to act mad or feign anger but all I could do was laugh. He can be a funny little bastard when he wants to be.

Being the current primary bread winner in the house, my husband often forgets about many of the symptoms of lupus such as fatigue. I honestly don't think he's being mean or evil. He actually forgets. There are times when we tribe members look just fine so why would our significant others remember that fatigue is one of the primary symptoms of lupus. Why, dear God, would they remember that standing over the stove can be a challenge when your hips hurt? Some folks don't mean any harm, they just ain't too bright.

The only thing he sees is that he's getting up five days a week, going to work to make money to support his family while I'm sitting at home watching daytime television, doing jack shit. Doesn't he know that since All My Children went off the air there's nothing left worth watching?

We've been living like this for a couple years now and at the beginning, I felt really bad for him. I worked for a PR firm in Washington, DC for over 18 years. I worked as long as I could. I've paid my dues; it's his turn.

We are, for all intents and purposes, a normal American family. Maybe I should say, African American family but we don't make that kind of money. Therefore, we're black people. I guess if we were a sitcom, we'd be a combination of the Bunkers and the Huxtables. We love our kids but we are definitely not the PC type of family. Personally, I think that being politically correct can work against you when raising kids.

Growing up in the 70's, I learned good old fashioned, real family values. My father was wonderful at saying what he meant and meaning what he said. We understood the poor guy perfectly. I remember being a very small child and hearing my father lovingly chastise my brother by hollering, "if you don't get your dumb-ass out the street, a car is going to hit you and the neighbors are going to laugh at you." See. It's easy. He didn't take 15 minutes out of his life to go into the street, kneel in front of this young lad and say something stupid like, "didn't we talk about safety first?"

Oh no. Not that guy. Daddy added many years to his life by simply being honest. As for our mother, she was a different breed altogether. If you're over 35, you'll understand when I say you haven't truly lived unless you've tasted gold, ducked a hair brush or learned a new word while weeping.

My first true learning experience with my mother happened at the grocery store. I'm holding my mother's hand as we are shopping. She selects the groceries and I stand on my tip toes and drop the food into the cart. It's simple and fun. Suddenly, one of our neighbors comes around the corner and they begin to gossip. I started out polite, quiet and respectful – or so I thought.

My mom starts recanting the story of what happened to us on the way to the store. Some idiot cut us off coming into the parking lot. I immediately speak up to correct her by saying, "no he didn't. You cut him off."

She looks at me and says, "Hada, be quiet." Warning number one. Then she starts to tell about how she called the guy an idiot. I say, "no you didn't, You called him a bad word." Mommy looked at me with a strange stare and said, "I'm not going to tell you again. Shut up."

Wow. How rude, right? Well now I'm embarrassed. It was the 70s and parents didn't come down to your height and whisper in your ear. Her point was clear. Me parent, you child, enough said. This was officially warning number two.

They moved on to another subject like who didn't give back a Tupperware bowl after a game of Pinochle. Something way over my head but I'm bored and obviously had short term memory loss back then.

We're all walking together and as we get to the back of the store where they kept the milk, my mother said, not to me of course, "I can't believe how high these prices are getting. We're going to starve at this rate," and that's where I fucked up. I immediately, without skipping a beat said, "but daddy said he got a raise so we can..." WHACK. Gold. Tears.

Did my mother lean down to pick me up or comfort me? Did she have even the slightest look of embarrassment on her face? Oh, no. This broad rose up to her full height and said slowly and clearly, "come here." I got up and walked to where she was standing and she hit me with a look I had never seen before and said, "Don't you ever contradict me in public again." A splendid educational moment with my mother and the word of the day was contradict.

I'm about to do the 5 year old scream when I hear her say, "cut all that noise out and put this in the cart before I give you something to cry about. What flavor ice cream do you want?" Like nothing happened.

Parents back then didn't have a reason to negotiate. They did the best they could and didn't owe us a damn thing. You knew what you did and you knew what you owed. I'm pretty sure I got butter pecan that day.

What does any of this have to do with lupus? Who knows? Maybe it was all the heavy metals (gold) I consumed as a child that caused this condition. Keep it simple. I was illustrating the values that we have passed down to our precious morons. The first major lesson I taught my kids was simply never to shame me in the street. Second, don't shame your family if you can avoid it. The middle child never quite got that one down, bless her heart.

My husband spent most of his time trying to make them clean the house, pick up wet clothes off the bathroom floor and checking behind them to make sure they turn the lights off when they leave a room because electricity costs money. Poor fool. And their favorite was when he insisted that they not let the water run in the sink while doing the dishes because water costs money.

One evening, it was our sons turn to do the dishes and he patiently waited for his father to come home so he could prove what a wonderful listener he was. My son was about 12 years old at the time and all of our kids have vivid imaginations and marvelous senses of humor.

I heard the kids whispering earlier in the evening but didn't really think anything of it. Hell, they were always scheming about something. It was us against them and they sometimes won. Their favorite rule in our house was if it's funny, you might actually get away with it.

So on this night he waits for his father to get home and sit down at the dining room table which, by the way, was in clear view of the kitchen sink.

My husband sits down and starts the whole 'how was your day, is your homework done' speech as our son goes into the kitchen to do the dishes. This boy begins to lick individual dishes, wipe them with a dish towel and put them in the cabinet like its normal procedure.

Not to be outdone, sisters then come behind him and start licking the glasses. Before my poor husband could catch himself he stands up and hollers, "what the fuck are you doing," and the girls and I break out into hysterical laughter. We're all about to pee on the floor because of his knee-jerk reaction and verbal faux pau. In a very leveled tone my brilliant son says, "we're trying to wash the dishes without letting the water run. Don't you know that water costs money?"

Cost of dishes: $25

Cost of dish towels: $5

The look on my husband's face: priceless

My husband begins to stomp towards the bedroom, but as he's leaving, he shouts, "now I have an entire houseful of assholes." One of the girls, with tears of laughter running down her face, testified that he also said, "I hate y'all." The rest of us were laughing too hard to hear that part.

Having lupus has given me an insight I didn't think I'd have until I was 70. It often allows me to see things as they really are and not worry about the small stuff. My position at this point is similar to the plaque I have hanging at my front door. It says, an unkempt house is better than a life unlived.

It's like when you have your first child. This is your precious baby and you are going to be the perfect parent. You sterilize everything. You make sure that visitors wash their hands before touching this holy child. You use only bottles that don't seep toxins and diapers that will prevent diaper rash. You might breast feed and hold the baby up properly to feed it. Some of us even bought changing tables, diaper holders and child approved laundry detergent. Let's not even talk about the special baby food we buy for this child. We go all out.

The second child makes you feel the same way but you learn to tone it down a bit. You learn that it's okay to lick the pacifier if it falls on the floor. Hot soapy water will work when washing bottles so you've never really pulled out the sterilizer. You throw dirty diapers into the trash can and you change the baby on the bed, floor or wherever you happen to be at the time. You still hum to the precious baby but the lullaby might change and the diapers are not as expensive. You actually wait for the diaper to be wet or muddy to change this kid and poop ain't as cute as it used to be. This child can miraculously eat soft table food and we begin to use our blenders more because we know it's just as good and less expensive.

Child number three and beyond is screwed. These little bastards are allowed to juggle knives if it keeps him or her from screaming. You give the bottles a good rinse. As long as there's no visible dog shit on your visitor's hands or clothes you pass the child off gladly and try to hide.

If this precious child should drop the pacifier in the middle of the night, you simply dip it into your glass of bourbon, and give it back and never miss a moment of The Nightly Show. You may never admit it to another living soul but you learned that propping a bottle on a pillow and letting them fall to sleep with it is not going to ruin them for life.

You'll know these children on sight. They are the ones with hand-me-down clothes, walking around in a circle on the playground singing, "nobody knows the trouble I've seen…nobody knows my sorrow."

If there is no smoke, blood or exposed bone, there's no reason to panic. Stress + Lupus = Very Bad.

That's where I am. I don't panic anymore. Three of our children are officially grown and out of the nest and the last one is being prepped to not only leave our home in four years but to leave joyfully. This, fellow lupus tribe members is a trick we learned with child number one. Start placing major demands on them at 16 and by 18 you're in the clear.

Times have changed and if you don't prepare now, they'll be living in your basement, trying to steal your medical marijuana and telling you how to run your home. Rent will be a dirty word and they'll always come up short or try to make you feel guilty about paying their share of the electric and water bill. Didn't their father tell them, "these things cost money?"

I think our son is afraid and who could blame him. You try growing up in a house with all girls and see how you feel. My heart went out to him. How much PMS can a guy take? He was really thrilled to get the hell out. Actually the girls were not as happy to see him go. I think he was exacting revenge when he would leave the toilet seat up at midnight. By 7:00 am, there would inevitably be a splash and scream and he would giggle happily. It was funny so…

We are a blended family. I didn't meet my step-son until he was 11. I remember this really shy, little kid with a baseball hat standing on a porch waiting to be picked up. He was adorable and has been mine ever since. Not that we don't know he's an ungrateful savage like his siblings, its' just that he's our only male ungrateful savage and we're a little protective.

The kids forged their relationship in the first 5 minutes of meeting each other. I told them to be nice to him because he was shy but what is the first thing the middle girl said to him?" "You look stupid in that hat." First impressions and all that. So yeah, leaving the toilet seat up was fine with me. I think the first thing I said to him was, "welcome, young man, to Clown University where you will learn the fine arts of sarcasm and idiocy." He was an excellent student.

Lupus can be a handy tool when you have kids. When you're having a lupus day and they want to talk with you about things that don't matter like Lady Gaga wearing a meat dress to the awards show, or who said what to whom. You can fake too tired to deal or you can say "are you intentionally trying to kill me?"

The last time I said it, Ms. 13 said, "yeah, but not today." She's such a smart-ass.

Okay, maybe I over used the 'I'm tired' routine. Most of the time it's not a lie and I really am tired. I find it to be very effective. Another way to get them from harassing you is to immediately pull out your medication bottles and begin to count out your pills while they babble.

I don't mind saying what I know you're thinking. One day, these people are going to dump my ass into the 'After All I've Done for You' Nursing Home and Supper Club, so what the hell.

Children

We all have a favorite something. Car, ice cream, beer, but my favorite something right now is a person. It's my three year old grandson, Jay. Notice how he gets name recognition and the others get numbers? Well, Jay understands me better than any of our children.

He is mildly autistic so he doesn't speak well yet nor is he potty trained. Nope, dude just doesn't have time for bullshit. He comes into the house and does his thing. We laugh, he gives me big hugs and the thing that I love the most is that if I'm down stairs too long, he'll take my hand and start walking me up the stairs.

He places me on the bed where he thinks I should be, gives me a toy to play with (usually his Fisher Price dump truck) and leaves me alone. When I'm not down stairs when he gets here, he comes up to look for me. He's the one who makes sure I'm healthy by sharing a juice box with me – I'm not hard to please.

Jay understands that I need to rest. His aunts and mother are jealous and say hateful things like, "well that's where you always are so he thinks that where you belong. He see's you there so much that he associates your bed with you."

No! Our love cannot be summed up in those terms. They are vile and filled with jealousy. He loves me and wants me to be well so that I can take him to the zoo. He's my main man.

I miss hanging out with my children. When the older kids were young we did all kinds of things. I would take them to museums on the weekend. We live in Washington, DC and everything is free. If it was free, we were there. My poor baby – the last of our brood didn't go many places with me because either, my body hurt, it was too hot, I was having a bad day, it was too sunny, my uterus was falling out. If I was having a good day, we just up and went. And if something really cool was happening, I would call one of her siblings and offer them cash. One does what one can.

You can get almost anything you want if gas money is offered.

Employment

I developed Graves disease and lost my mind. If you know anything about thyroid disorders you know what I'm talking about. Lupus + thyroid disorder = functional lunatic. It was so bad that one day I thought I was having a stroke. My heart started pounding, I broke into a sweat, I got dizzy and could not breathe. My face went numb, the whole nine yards. This all happened in my office while I was trying to format a press release.

Anyway I'm trying to get myself together without screaming at the top of my lungs, 'pimp down! pimp down!' and finally my body begins to respond. I said my body, not my brain. I tried to ignore what I was feeling and pushed the send button for my press release. The lesson I learned was never try to work while you are impaired. I'm sure they called me all kinds of stupid but I couldn't help it.

Parts of my body would suddenly seize up while I was at work and I'd try to stay in my office as much as possible. For about a month I was having problems with my arms and they would ache if I didn't hold them in a certain way, so I was walking around the office looking crazy. One of my coworkers told me one day that I should not hold my arms that way because I look stupid. It was cool because he was and still is one of my dearest friends. But it let me know that people were probably talking about me.

Discoid lupus is my primary diagnosis so of course I spent years trying to hide my hair loss but there was nothing I could do about my SLE or my skin discoloration and scars. Wearing makeup burned my skin and exacerbated the condition, so I only used it when we had our annual Christmas party. Any other time I looked and felt like the office monster.

I remember the day I went into my boss's office and handed him my resignation. I remember being in such unbelievable physical and emotional pain. I don't remember if I cried or not but I wanted to. I didn't tell him about the pain but I talked about dumb mistakes I had made and how sorry I was. He treated me more like a father then an employee and let me know it was okay and that he 'got it.' Hell, he even offered me a sabbatical but even then I knew that this condition would progress and we'd one day end up in the same office having the same conversation.

For tribe members who are employed, I feel confident that you know of what I speak. Particularly if you loved your job like I did. We had a blast. I can't even begin to tell you how much I miss it.

If you are the sole bread winner in your home, do the best you can but don't kill yourself over it. We'll talk later on about options that might help. I'm convinced I worked three years too long and pushed myself a step too far.

Money

Sound Check: *If Trouble Were Money*
Soundtrack: *Jason's Lyric, Mint Condition*

While I'm writing this, I can honestly say that I'm so poor I can't even pay attention. I'm broke as a bag of glass. I don't answer my home phone anymore I'm tired of saying, "Jimmy no live here" with a Mexican accent.

The issue of money will eventually come up during your visit to lupus land so prepare yourself. You and your significant other could find yourselves standing in the middle of the floor saying, "bust a move." I told my husband when I started writing that I'm donating a portion of the proceeds from this book to the Lupus Foundation of America.

You would have thought I told him I was selling one of his daughters into prostitution. This man goes ballistic and begins to, again, tell me every single thing his money pays for, how he works so hard to keep a roof over our heads, blah, blah, gas bill, electric bill, blah, blah, my wine supply (wink). It sounded like a super villain monologue. I got mad and told him that since he feels that way about it, I'm giving it all to them. I think he had a minor stroke because his eyes rolled to the back of his head and he was rendered speechless. I didn't even look at the phone; least of all reach for it. Die dog! Seriously though, he works his ass off to support us and I love him for it.

Unless you're extremely wealthy, all couples argue about money at some point or another. I've always been the primary bread winner so for my husband, this is relatively new and unpleasant.

I know that any of my dear, personal friends who are reading this are rolling around on the floor in tears, laughing. Y'all cut it out. Breathe, Mikki…breathe. See our money situation has always been a little, ah, tumultuous so for my husband to get upset seems a bit irrational to our friends. Mikki, get off the floor and go get your inhaler, okay? I can hear you wheezing from here. Excuse her, tribe. She can be down-right rude sometimes.

The vast majority of us know how to deal with money issues because we learned as children. Remember during that 105 degree heat wave when your dad came home and shouted, "turn this goddamn air conditioner off!" You remember it. It was on the same day your mom appeared from out of the kitchen with her six shooter in hand and you could hear her spurs make that clinging sound on the floor as she sashayed ever so slowly towards the window unit. The tumble weed rolled across the room between them. Do you remember the look in her eyes as she stood wide legged with her trusty pistol pointed squarely at his head? I remember the words that she spoke as though they were gospel. "Ya feelin' lucky, punk?"

My father's response was brilliant. He simply said, "No. But tell your dumb-ass son to get out of the street before he gets hit by a car," and walked away. Yeah, they were having cash flow problems at the time.

Money issues can be very tricky. On the one hand you either feel guilty about your condition and being unable to work or you feel like your resources (disability, part-time pay check, whatever) aren't enough. On the other hand, your spouse leaves home every day, comes home dog tired and often feeling defeated and at the end of the month. There are months that you barely have enough money to meet the mortgage. My lights are blinking as we speak.

Be loving towards each other. It's a bummer for all involved when T-bones on the gas grill turn into burgers in the frying pan. But you have each other and at the end of the day, what's more important. So what you had to give up cable in order to eat. You don't need to sit up all night watching *HBO.* Have sex instead or talk about why you're not having sex.

Like lupus, everyone's circumstance is different. You've got to find what works for you and hopefully, you will have that happy ending you see in movies. Either that or your girlfriend, Linda will loan you money and laugh at you because she can - Love you, girl!! Can I borrow $20 for old time sake?

Now pay attention because this bit is very important. Do not allow anyone to mistreat you. Unfortunately, our condition is too complicated for some people. They really did love us once but the intestinal fortitude it takes to care for us does not exist in everyone. It's sad and we try to give them space and time but sometimes it is all for naught.

Sound Check: *I can't make you love me if you don't*
Soundtrack: *Bonnie Raitt*

NOT FUNNY, OR PREPARE
FOR THE F-BOMB

(you choose a title)

Sound Check: *Lowrider by War*

I've been thinking about how to go about this. I'm seriously pissed off and don't have the energy or wherewithal to even attempt to be polite but I will try.

If you have lupus, I suspect you're angry as hell and we have every right. Be outraged, scream at your congress person, yell obscenities at your physician (that's always fun). Do what you need to do to be heard. You can do what I did and call the lupus foundation and say to whomever answers the phone, "what the fuck!?"

I mean as soon as they say hello. Actually, that's how I met one of my best friends because when she said hello, I did my what the fuck thing and she started to laugh and said, true story, "I don't know but you might wanna cut back on the prednisone?" You go V!! Be bold.

Not to begrudge any other person with a life threatening or chronic illness but I gotta let you know that our tribe always seems to get the shitty end of the stick.

For example: Cancer patients have access to new trial drugs and medication almost every other year. They are creating wonderful vaccines that can possibly alleviate breast, prostate, brain, fill in the blank _____ cancers or at the very least, extend life expectancy. I sincerely believe it's a wonderful thing. They have access to wigs, cosmetics, clothes, support groups everywhere and thousands of people walk to raise money for the cause every 6 months.

HIV/AIDS. I remember during the 80's when positive meant death. When there was so much shame and stigma attached to the virus that most people didn't even want to talk about it. It was a hush, hush disease. When you think about catching hell, think of them. I remember taking my children to see the AIDS quilt when it came to DC. Their favorite aunt who has since passed away died because of the disease. I sympathize with them all.

We marched, ran marathons, partnered with a few patients just to help them get out of bed in the morning. I actually encouraged both of my girls to work with me at the food bank twice a week because they needed to understand that everyone with HIV is not gay or a bad person or any of the labels society was/is placing on them.

Having said all that, you know that I'm not just whining or being a brat – though I did kind of lay on the floor kicking and screaming earlier.

Think about it. Remember what I said earlier. Other groups get help from all over the world. They have wigs made free of charge and people donate their hair for this. For cancer patients who have chemo scars, there is makeup to help cover the burns. Come to think about it, so do burn victims. There is a support group around every corner in major cities that have regular meetings where people get together and discuss what's going on in their lives and how happy or angry they are. Medical trials out the wazoo. People who volunteer to go to homes and help with the basic day to day 'stuff.' Help with shopping, laundry, you name it.

What do we have? Jack Shit!! There are people with lupus who can't bathe or dress themselves. People who because of this disease, can't hold a pen or even answer the phone if it rings. They need support. Those of us who know about these people try to do what we can, but unlike the cancer society and AIDS network, there is no official list of who needs this help. Some of them are suicidal – been there, done that – but are in too much pain to get to the pharmacy and pick up a simple anti-depressant med so they can O.D. The pain is both physical and emotional. We fucking hurt.

If you've been able to read this far then you know that lupus is chronic and in most cases, progressive. It tends to mask itself as other conditions like renal failure, heart disease, thyroid disease, etc. But for our tribe the underlying case is SLE. You feelin' me, right?

Why then, has it taken 50 years to come up with a new lupus drug that actually works? I'm sorry. Maybe you didn't hear me so let me say it differently. 50 FUCKING YEARS!! That means there has not been a decent medication for lupus since before I was born. How sad is that? In my mind, it's criminal. The best medication we have (or so they say) is called Plaquenil. It was originally designed to cure malaria. Yes, that's what I said – MALARIA. Show of hands here: who knows anyone with lupus who has malaria? Seriously, think about it. I'll wait…

Yeah, yeah, I know there is a scientific reason why this drug works for both diseases. Thank you, wonderful, caring physicians for recommending a drug that will allow us to fly over to Bangkok (I love that name) and party with our friends without getting a dreaded case of malaria (hear harsh sarcasm) and being able to cure that tiny, little case of syphilis we'll most likely come home with. Ungrateful, you say? Damn skippy, but let's talk about why I feel this way.

50 years to the average person is a long fucking time. For our tribe, it's more than our life expectancy. We are dying from this disease. Plaquenil may actually work but after getting pissed off again and doing some research, I found out that plaquenil only truly helps about 1/3 of the people who have this debilitating disease. The only thing it does for me is give me a splitting headache.

Recently, I spoke to a young woman at the opticians office (gotta get that damn vision field test every six months while you're on plaquenil) and she said her mother had just died of lupus in June. First of all, I was speechless because she didn't know me, had never seen me before but recognized the butterfly rash on my face. The more we talked, the more my heart broke for her. She was only 18 years old. Her mother, after years of having missed school performances, parent teacher conferences, amusement parks and the like, raised herself out of her bed to be at her daughters high school graduation and passed away 3 days later.

My teenage daughter was in the room while this young woman was telling me her story. Usually, my kids face is lowered into her iPod or cell phone keypad so I know she's not paying attention to this conversation. When we left the opticians office, as we were walking towards the car, my daughter took my hand and whispered to me, "please don't die." Needless to say, we got into the car and kind of lost it for a few minutes. When we were finished crying, I called her stupid and went home. I didn't miss my turn that day either.

Hmmm, what to do.

Please indulge me while make a few suggestions or go off on a personal diatribe. Before I do, I need to make it perfectly clear that I AM, IN NO WAY SHAPE OR FORM, SPEAKING FOR OR ON BEHALF OF THE LUPUS FOUNDATION. Please don't send them nasty letters about something I said that rubbed you the wrong way. They are doing the best they can with what they have to work with and it ain't much. It's not like the government is handing them stacks of cash for research.

Doctors, physicians, whatever you prefer to be called, get a grip. Stop being scared of this disease and become part of our solution. Quit passing the buck. I'm convinced that had the first seven doctors I went to with mystery symptoms, that made some half-hearted comment about something called a butterfly rash had actually ordered blood work that included an ANA, I might have been treated sooner. Big shout out to the one that admitted that it might be out of her league and referred me to the dermatologist who actually did a skin biopsy and got the ball rolling.

It's a scary disease. It can present like an ordinary cold sometimes but how many colds can one person have in a year? Think about it. Your patient is telling you how fatigued he/she feels. They are telling you how hard it is to get up in the morning and function. How they are suddenly having moments of memory loss. On and on. Is it too much to ask that you do a thorough check of this person's immune system? I mean, really? You just send them home with an omega three and once a day vitamin suggestion? Really?!

It's not entirely your fault and I know that. I know that you've got to go through the insurance company and follow hospital procedure or lose your license. However, would it really hurt to do what some of the older, more experienced doctors do? Tell a teeny tiny little white lie. Beef it up just enough to get the testing approved. Who's going to know? You won't miss a moment of sleep if it helps to save a life. Remember, do no harm. Sometimes inaction can cause more harm than good. I'm just saying…

Insurance companies, wow. What to say? Oh, I know… screw you! I know you've heard it before but I really gotta say it to get if off my heart. Screw you! Screw you in your stupid, money grubbing, self-interested, pig asses. For the record, I'm talking 'squeal like a pig', dueling banjos, white water rafting, screwed by an inbred mongrel type screw.

We are suffering. We are dying. Why do you need for my epitaph to read "died of red tape and bullshit?" Why do you need for my family to file a lawsuit after I'm dead, when all you needed to do was approve me for a damn drug that nine times out of ten would have kept me alive? I can't talk about this anymore. I fucking hate you! I need a drink. OMFG!

There have been celebrities that have spoken up about lupus. Richard Dryfuss, Julian Lennon, Will and Jada Smith. Believe it or not, the list keeps growing every day. Just recently, Nick Canon was diagnosed with this disease and spoke publicly at a Lupus gala. Welcome to the tribe, my brother.

My problem with this is that it's all done at Gala's that I can't afford to attend. Beyond that, all I have to say is, "thank you." Thank you from the bottom of my heart. Thank you for your time, your dollars, your love the whole shebang. Please keep speaking up for us.

For the rest of you, I'll keep it simple. We need you, too. I've been to enough holiday work gatherings and company get togethers to know that you truly are a charitable group. Big shout out. During my employment with, not sure if I can say their name, so I'll just call it the PR firm, we did serious charity work on the side. Remember hurricane Katrina? We collected and purchased so much stuff that we needed to make more than three trips to the drop off center.

We collected new and gently used books and donated them to organizations like The Hospital for Sick Children. Y'all, the list goes on and on.

Our church donates generously, to the homeless efforts and anything else one of our members or non-members need.

We all know those kinds of people and places. I suspect you do as well, so here's what I'd like for you to do this year. This year at your holiday party, have a fund raiser for Lupus. Put it on your invitations so that people will know and have check, cash or money orders already written out. I'd love to be more polite about it and sound all cute a fuzzy but I don't have time. This disease might kill me and will definitely kill many of my tribe members before the end of the year. That more than anything makes my wolf really angry.

Trust me. If you need someone to come and explain why you're doing this or be a lupus rep, we will be there with no hesitation. I'll come – with or without makeup and thank everyone personally. Beware, pioneer!!! If you work for an insurance company, you really don't want me there but I can find you someone else who doesn't hate you as much. I'm sorry but I have a family and can't afford to go all Charles Bronson and end up in jail.

Students, we really need you guys too. You all were more than influential in getting Obama elected. I know you can do this thing. Hold a few rally's every year. I'll come. I've been to Hood College, UMD and several more and I've seen your enthusiasm. You, young people, are unbelievable assets to any cause or charity. We need that kind of enthusiasm in order to stay alive.

Don't wait for one of your student body to be diagnosed before you start screaming. We should all be screaming. We should all be outraged. I'm not the only one who should be mad as hell. We should all be angry wolves. ROAR!!

Sound Check: *Never Give Up by Yolanda Adams*

Printed in the United States
By Bookmasters